Intermittent Fasting for Women Over 50

A Complete Guide to Lose Weight, Get Fit, Eat Healthy with a 21 Day Meal Plan

Nancy Vassallo

Copyright © 2023 by Nancy Vassallo - All rights reserved.

Table of Contents

INTRODUCTION

In the last several years, there have been many food fads, but the essential medical advice on what makes a healthy lifestyle has remained relatively unchanged: consume foods that are low in fat, increase the amount of activity you get, and under no circumstances miss meals.

Yet, during the same period, obesity rates have skyrocketed throughout the globe. Is there thus an alternative strategy supported by evidence? One founded on evidence rather than personal opinion?

We believe that there is.

Intermittent Fasting

When we first heard about the supposed health advantages of intermittent fasting, we, along with many other people, had our doubts.

Going without food for an extended period sounded extreme and challenging, and we were both aware that dieting, in any form, is almost always guaranteed to fail.

However, after doing in-depth research on it and putting it to use ourselves, we are confident of the extraordinary potential it has.

There is nothing else you can do to your body that is as powerful as fasting.

In ancient times and in current times, people have used fasting as a tactic.

The human body was built to go without food for extended periods. We are the result of millennia of feast and famine; our evolution occurred during a period when food was in short supply. Because the environment in which contemporary humans were formed is replicated significantly more exactly by intermittent fasting than by eating three meals a day, this may be why we react so well to the practice of intermittent fasting.

The practice of fasting continues to be deeply ingrained in many people's religious beliefs. Some of the most famous examples are the fasts observed during the seasons of Lent, Yom Kippur, and Ramadan.

According to Saint Nikolai of Zicha, "Gluttony makes a man gloomy and fearful, but fasting makes him joyful and courageous."

In addition, Greek Orthodox Christians are urged to fast for 180 days out of the year, but Buddhist monks fast on the new moon and full moon of each lunar month.

However, it seems that more of us are eating most of the time. We seldom, if ever, feel the need to eat. However, we are not content with this regarding our size, body, and state of health. We can reconnect with our human selves via the practice of intermittent fasting.

It is a path that leads to a reduction in body fat and improved health and well-being over the long term.

Scientists have just scratched the surface to discover and demonstrate how potent a tool it can be.

The Fast Diet

> We are aware that the conventional wisdom on how one should eat does not work for many individuals.
>
> The Fast Diet offers a radical new approach. It can revolutionize how we think about food and how to get rid of excess weight.

The Fast Diet requires considering what we consume and the timing of those meals.

However, the technique is adaptable, easy to understand, and user-friendly, and there are no too burdensome restrictions to adhere to.

➢ There is no daily drudgery of calorie restriction, none of the boredom, irritation, or repeated deprivation that characterizes traditional diet regimes, and so on.

➢ Yes, it requires fasting, but not in the traditional sense; you won't "starve" on any day if you follow this method.

You won't have to stretch up any of the meals you like. In the majority of instances

➢ Once the weight has been lost, continuing with the basic regimen will ensure that it remains lost if you do so.

➢ One of the benefits of following the Fast Diet is reducing body weight. However, the actual payoff comes in possible long-term health improvements, such as a reduced risk of various ailments such as diabetes, cardiovascular disease, and cancer.

➢ You will quickly realize that it is more than simply a diet, and I say this with all sincerity. It is much more than that: it is a long-term plan for maintaining good health and living a whole life.

The Logic Behind Science

In the wild, most animals go through cycles of feasting and starvation as a natural part of their lives.

Our distant ancestors did not typically have four or five meals every day.

Instead, they would kill, gorge themselves, and then just laze about for a while before being forced to go for extended stretches without anything to eat.

Our bodies and our genes were shaped by an environment of deprivation, which was interspersed with the occurrence of periodic catastrophic events.

Things are not similar as they were in the past at all.

We never seem to stop eating. People often see fasting, which consists of voluntarily refraining from consuming meals, as an odd practice, not to mention one that is detrimental to one's health.

Most of us anticipate consuming at least three meals per day and ample snacks between those meals.

In addition to the meals and the snacks, we also eat throughout the day.

This can consist of a creamy cappuccino here, a unique cookie, or even a smoothie since it is considered "healthier."

Once upon a time, parents cautioned their offspring against snacking between mealtimes hours. Those days are a distant memory at this point. Recent research conducted in the United States found that the amount of time spent between what the researchers cheekily described as 'eating occasions' has decreased by one hour.

The study compared the eating behaviors of 28,000 children and 36,000 adults over the last thirty years. To put it another way, over the past several decades, the amount of time we spend "not eating" has significantly decreased.

In the 1970s, adults such as my mother would go around four and a half hours without eating, while the average expectation for youngsters like myself was that we could go approximately four hours without eating.

The time has been cut down to three and a half hours for adults and three hours for youngsters, and this does not include any beverages or snacks.

The notion that eating less often but more frequently is a "good thing" has roots in the popular diet book industry and snack food marketing, but it has also received backing from the mainstream medical community.

They argue that eating several smaller meals throughout the day is preferable since doing so reduces the likelihood that we would get hungry and then binge on high-fat junk food.

I can see where you're coming from, and some studies show there may be some health advantages to eating smaller meals more often, but, to reap those benefits, you can't just wind up consuming more food overall.

Unfortunately, the unfortunate truth is that such a thing occurs in the real world.

According to the findings of the study that I cited earlier, not only do we consume an additional 180 calories per day in snacks, the majority of which come in the form of milky and fizzy drinks as well as smoothies, but we also consume an additional 120 calories per day during our regular meals.

This represents a significant increase in our overall caloric intake.

Put another way, it would seem that snacking does not result in less food being consumed at mealtimes; rather, it only whets the hunger.

LOSING WEIGHT WITH INTERMITTENT FASTING

It is one of the popular and successful methods that I've employed in my practice to support the weight-loss objectives of my clients.

I've found that it helps my clients lose weight more quickly and effectively.

This chapter will discuss what intermittent fasting is, why it is effective, and why I am so convinced that once you begin, you will wonder why you waited so long to give it a try and wonder what took you so long to give it a try.

What exactly does it mean to "fast" intermittently?

The practice of deliberately extending or shortening the time during which a person goes without food is known as intermittent fasting.

This kind of fasting falls under the more general category of intermittent fasting.

You could decide to engage in intermittent fasting for some reasons, including the desire to simplify your life, satisfy particular lifestyle preferences, improve your health, or reduce your body fat percentage.

These are the two most fundamental concerns raised by intermittent fasting:

1. How long does it take you from the first bite of food you eat one day to the first mouthful of food you eat the following day?

2. Would you be willing to make that time frame longer? How often and by what amount? Your responses will determine what intermittent fasting means to you, and what it means to you is likely to change over time as you gain more experience, become more self-aware, and mature.

The majority of variations of intermittent fasting do not stipulate what kinds of foods you are permitted or forbidden to consume; instead, you are tasked with giving more significant consideration to the order in which you take your meals on any given day.

The recipes supplied in part 2 have been carefully created to direct you toward a healthy way of eating; yet, they will not artificially limit you from consuming any food category.

Changing the directive in which you eat your meals could improve your health, but would this be a significant change?

Both history and contemporary scientific research share this view. In human history, many different kinds of intermittent fasting have been practiced by various cultures for various reasons, including those related to medicine and religion.

Some courageous individuals even attempt prolonged fasts, which consist of going without meals for a lengthy period (usually several days). These kinds of fasts are pretty strenuous, and although a tiny percentage of individuals may find them enjoyable, the vast majority of people do not find them all that attractive.

They are not required to reap the advantages that are connected with fasting. As a result, lengthy fasts that last for many days are not covered in this book.

Instead, we will focus on six daily and weekly intermittent fasting; each includes fasts that may last somewhere from 12 to 24 hours in length. Let's take a more in-depth look at the choices we have.

VARIATIONS ON THE THEME OF INTERMITTENT FASTING

This section will better understand the various types of intermittent fasting options available to you.

In addition, this will explain the differences between daily and weekly fasts and the subtypes that fall under these two main categories of fasting schedules.

My approach to advising customers who are interested in fasting on the sort of intermittent fast that is most suitable for them follows a straightforward philosophy, which is as follows: We modify fasting to accommodate your lifestyle rather than rearranging your life to accommodate fasting.

Put another way, you do not need to completely upend both your personal and professional life to conform to an arbitrary diet plan.

On the contrary, it is expected that fasting would make your life less complicated and more joyful.

FASTS DONE ON A DAILY OR NEARLY DAILY BASIS

Fasts done daily or nearly daily are referred to as fasts done daily.

The number designations refer to the time window during which one must consume food or refrain from doing so.

Those who are new to fasting or wish to ease into it can do any of the daily fasts listed below on alternate days rather than every day, as they see appropriate. This is entirely up to them.

12:12

The 12:12 fast is the most minimalistic form of the intermittent fasting technique. On this fast, allow a 12-hour buffer from your final bite one day to your first bite the following day.

For instance, if you finish eating at seven o'clock in the evening, you may have your next meal at seven o'clock in the morning.

This fast is a great initial entry point for individuals concerned about how they might respond to intermittent fasting or those who are not yet interested in going without food for more than 12 hours.

In addition, it serves as an excellent starting point for those who are not yet interested in fasting for longer than 12 hours.

16:8

The 16:8 method of fasting is the one that is used by the majority of people.

This fast designates an eight-hour "eating window" that begins 16 hours after the final food of one day and continues until the first bite of the next day.

For instance, if you finish eating at seven in the evening, you may have your next meal at eleven in the morning. It is an upfront and logical process that may be eased into utilizing a 14:10 kind of fasting as an intermediate step if that is what the individual who is doing the fasting decides they would want to do.

ONE MEAL A DAY (OMAD)

One meal a day, often known as OMAD, is a simplified method of describing a fast that is ultimately similar to a 22:2, 23:1, or even 24:0 fast.

You would have a single, substantial meal after going at least 22 hours without eating anything in this fast.

For example, if you finished eating one night at seven o'clock, you would probably wait a whole day before eating again, and you would probably eat between five and seven o'clock in the evening. It is more probable that the OMAD method of fasting will be utilized more dynamically — once in a while — rather than as a firm and consistent guideline to follow every day.

This is considered a more challenging version of the daily fast.

WEEKLY FASTS

The difference between a weekly fast and a daily fast is that you may only be obliged to abstain from food for a few days of the week.

However, you may be expected to pay somewhat more attention to the number of calories you consume on those days.

Of course, that depends on the approach you decide to take, so let's take a more in-depth look at the available choices, which increases the difficulty level.

In the 5:2 fast, you usually eat for five days of the week and then fast for the other two days by restricting your calorie intake to anywhere between 500 and 800 each day.

These calories may be ingested in a single, substantial meal, or they can be split over two meals or snacks that are less in size.

Alternately, a softer variation of the 5:2 fast would entail following a regular diet for five days of the week, followed by a 16-hour fast two days of the week without restricting calories specifically. This version of the fast would be continued for two weeks.

ALTERNATE-DAY MODIFIED FASTING (ADMF)

ADMF, also known as alternate-day modified fasting, is a kind of modified fasting in which participants alternate between days in which they are permitted to eat anything they want and days in which they must restrict their caloric intake.

You would consume between 500 and 800 calories throughout one to two meals or snacks on calorie-controlled fasting days.

This may appear like a calorie-controlled variant of the 16:8 eating pattern.

However, it is a more complicated variant of the 5:2 fast since you end up fasting for three to four days per week rather than simply two days per week while adhering to a calorie restriction plan.

ALTERNATE-DAY FASTING (ADF) comprises a recurrent cycle in which one day is spent eating normally and the next day is spent fasting entirely.

Alternate-day fasting, also known as ADF or 1:1 fasting, is another name.

This particular method of abstaining from food will likely be presented in the book in its most complex and challenging form. It might be a more manageable form of the alternate-day fasting strategy that is becoming more popular.

BUSTING FASTING MYTHS

The rapid rise in the popularity of fasting in recent years has attracted the attention of some critics.

On the other hand, one article published in 2017 in the journal Annual Review of Nutrition said that "evidence suggests that intermittent fasting regimens are not harmful physically or mentally (i.e., in terms of mood) in healthy adults."

This section will set the record straight and provide the facts when it comes to some of the rumors surrounding intermittent fasting.

Myth number one: If you fast, you will go hungry. It is not the same as starving to going without food for a while between meals.

Starvation is a condition that may be scientifically characterized as occurring when your body has used up a significant portion of its fat and glycogen stores and resorts to using protein (or, to put it another way, muscle) as a fuel source.

Myth number two: If you fast, you won't get enough nutrition. If someone merely decides to start fasting on a whim without giving more thought to their typical eating pattern, there is a chance that they may not get enough of certain nutrients, which might have negative costs on their health. That won't happen to anybody who reads this book; as long as you comprehend the meals you are most likely to slip and account for items that compose those meals elsewhere in your day, the danger of nutritional deficiency in your diet is minimal. Again, that won't happen to anyone who reads this book.

Myth number three: If you fast, you will overeat when you break your fast. When you fast, you should be prepared for the possibility that you may wind up eating more substantial meals less often. However, if you consider the act of overeating from the standpoint of the number of calories consumed, it is pretty unlikely that it will take place during a fasting program that has been well-prepared.

Furthermore, according to a report issued in the Annual Review of Nutrition in 2017, weight reduction is allegedly possible with almost every intermittent fasting routine.

How Men and Women Fast Otherwise One of the fundamental tenets of the scientific theory behind intermittent fasting is that it puts the body in a state of mild stress. Still, it makes the body more resistant to stress in the long run. It's almost like a training routine for your metabolism if you want to think of it that way. While this continues to be of great interest to investigators, we are left to grapple with how to approach fasting as a potential stressor.

This is particularly correct when considering how men and women react differently to stress both psychologically and biologically, as was investigated in a study conducted in 2009 and published in the journal Endocrine Disorders. This study found that women tend to have higher circulating levels of the stress hormone cortisol than men.

However, cortisol is not the only hormone that varies significantly between males and females. Another essential factor that should be taken into account for women is how the practice of intermittent fasting affects their menstrual cycles. Data from the month of Ramadan, during which people traditionally abstain from food and drink, may help us answer this issue.

The holy month of Ramadan is a simulation of an intermittent daily fast that lasts between 12 and 16 hours and provides valuable lessons that may be applied to various forms of fasting. According to the findings of research directed during Ramadan in 2013 and published in the Iranian Journal of Reproductive Medicine, menstrual irregularities increased, particularly among women who fasted for 15 or more days. Before Ramadan, just one in ten of the participants reported menstrual irregularities, but throughout Ramadan, that number increased to three in ten. In light of these statistics, it is undeniably essential to consider those who have a previous record of menstrual irregularities. From a hormonal standpoint, a second Ramadan-based study published in 2014 in the journal Clinical and

Experimental Obstetrics and Gynecology discovered critical female hormones. This study was published in response to whether or not women experience changes in their hormone levels during the holy month of fasting. When all of the evidence is measured, there is no need for women to be afraid of intermittent fasting; nonetheless, it is recommended that they pay a little more attention than usual to how their bodies react to it.

WHO CAN FAST, AND WHO CAN'T?

The overwhelming bulk of the information gathered points to the fact that otherwise healthy individuals may safely observe a fast without risking their mental or physical health. Even though I've had experience with various degrees of intermittent fasting with individuals from various walks of life and dietary backgrounds, I do not believe that fasting is a solution that can be applied universally. Specific individuals can only feel at ease during shorter fasts, while others have no problem with the longer ones. Fasting is not something that others should be doing at all. If you are not seeing an improvement in your quality of life due to your fasting, you should reconsider your decision to continue doing it. Before beginning a fast, those who have medical issues, whether they are acute or chronic, should talk to their doctor. Even though fasting on and off during the day is usually always done to enhance one's health, there are circumstances in which doing so may be harmful or not a good idea.

Among them are the following: A disordered eating past is presented. People who have a history of disordered eating or food restriction may find that some kinds of intermittent fasting partly replicate or resemble restricted eating methods, which may set up alarm bells.

Pregnant/breastfeeding.

Women who are pregnant or nursing have greater caloric demands than other women and ensuring that they get sufficient nutrients is a concern for their health and their kids' health.

Underweight/undernourished.

Even while there are other benefits to intermittent fasting outside weight reduction, some patterns naturally lead to consuming fewer calories than others. Anyone underweight or who has nutritional deficiencies should not engage in the practice of fasting. Particular pharmaceuticals. Because the effectiveness of some drugs is dependent on the consumption of different quantities of food, people mustn't put fasting ahead of their regularly scheduled prescription intake unless they have first spoken with a medical expert.

Children and teens.

Young individuals are at a time of fast growth and development, and as a result, their calorie and nutritional requirements are very high. The routine incorporation of fasting regimens has the potential to conflict with those requirements.

How the Practice of Intermittent Fasting Contributes to Weight Loss Intermittent fasting is a novel strategy for weight reduction that gives advantages through two distinct pathways, namely practical and metabolic. This strategy is only suitable for those in good health, willing, and able to follow it.

THE PRACTICAL PATH

The concept that intermittent fasting is an innovative and comfortable approach to eating fewer calories underpins the practical application of the fasting strategy for weight reduction, which is based on the idea that intermittent fasting is a road to weight loss. Just since there is less time dedicated to eating, people who engage in a protracted and regular program of intermittent fasting will consume fewer calories than they were used to, simply because there is less time in the day dedicated to eating. When a shorter eating window is combined with more substantial and gratifying options, like the ones discussed in this book, the potential for weight loss is undoubtedly there.

This claim is confirmed by the results of research published in 2018 in the journal Nutrition and Healthy Aging. That study indicated that fasting led to a slight decrease in calorie consumption without the requirement to measure or monitor calorie consumption. According to the metabolic pathway, fasting may provide certain metabolic benefits that make it easier to shed excess pounds.

A rising quantity of data suggests that fasting for lengthy periods regularly has a metabolically favorable impact on humans, and an increasing corpus of research supports this theory.

Research published in the journal Rejuvenation Research in 2015 found that intermittent fasting may change the expression of genes associated with human metabolism and lifespan.

Confirming the long-term effects of such alterations will require additional research, but there is no denying that these effects are of great interest.

Multiple studies, including the one that was cited earlier, a review paper published in 2017 by the journal Behavioural Sciences, and a paper published in 2018 in Cell Metabolism, have demonstrated that intermittent fasting has either a unique effect on circulating insulin levels or an effect that is superior to insulin resistance when compared to "normal dieting." Your liver and muscle cells may become less likely to take up and absorb circulating sugars as you age, contributing to greater blood sugar levels. This is because insulin resistance can develop due to poor eating choices and natural aging. Insulin is a significant driver of fat cell accumulation, as stated in a report published in one of the journals published by the American Heart Association in 2005. This implies that greater circulating insulin levels may encourage an increase in fatty tissue and contribute to weight gain. Some scientists believe fasting offers additional weight loss benefits because it improves the efficiency of the mechanisms in your body that process energy. By depriving your body of food for an extended period, these mechanisms are forced to be more adaptable, leading to weight loss.

Even though further study in this field is required before definitive conclusions can be drawn, a phenomenon known as metabolic flexibility may contribute to the advantages of intermittent fasting.

WHAT CHANGES DO YOU NOTICE WHEN YOU STOP EATING?

When you go without food for an extended period, your metabolism goes through several modifications. The practice of fasting will be broken down into three parts for this section's explanation. We keep the explanations within those boundaries since nowhere in this book does it propose a type of fasting that necessitates lasting any longer than 24 to 36 hours without eating.

The first stage is the federal state. (the first three hours following the last meal)

Insulin is secreted due to increased blood glucose caused by your most recent meal. It becomes more problematic for your body to utilize fat as fuel, and instead, it turns to carbs that are readily accessible for either energy or storage.

Consuming more calories than one needs might lead to fat storage.

Phase 2: The Beginning of the Fasting State (3 to 18 hours after the last meal) Your insulin and blood sugar levels return to normal. Your body begins to draw its energy supply from the glycogen reserves in your liver. As more time passes, your body will begin to generate energy by metabolizing fat instead of glucose.

The third stage is the fasting state (18 to 36 hours after the last meal). As you go through stage 2, your metabolism starts to change such that it uses fat mainly as a fuel source. At the same time, the danger of muscle breakdown increases, particularly after the first 36-hour period.

A Look at Fasting and the Hormone That Causes Hunger Signaling molecules known as hormones are responsible for various alterations all across the body.

The beneficial effects of fasting on hormone levels represent a kind of extension of the metabolic path; however, the link between intermittent fasting and hormones goes beyond just insulin. Insulin is the hormone that moves glucose into your cells to be used as energy; however, the beneficial effects of fasting on hormone levels represent a sort of extension of the metabolic path.

Consider the hormone known as ghrelin, sometimes known as the "hunger hormone," which gets its name because it is closely linked to appetite and tends to reach its peak level just before eating. A somewhat more advanced variation of the 16:8 fasting regimen detailed in this book is the 18:6 fasting regimen, the subject of research published in 2019 in Obesity.

The researchers discovered that even though the ladies were taking part in a daily fast that lasted for many hours, their appetite levels fell, and their hunger levels were more consistent. The clincher is... Their levels of the hormone that controls hunger also decreased.

Even though fasting should theoretically make you hungrier in the short run, it could help you become more in tune with your body's cues about whether or not you are genuinely hungry in the intermediate term.

How the 21-Day Plan Can Help You Achieve Your Weight-Loss Objectives The practice of intermittent fasting is a beneficial tool that may propel you forward on the road toward achieving your objectives; but, to assure success, it must be wisely utilized in combination with a nutritious diet.

HEALTHIER EATING WHILE FASTING

Your guide to maintaining a healthy diet while on a fast will be the 21-day schedule and the delicious dishes included in part 2.

The recipes adhere to a "clean eating" philosophy, emphasizing essential components of a healthy diet such as fruits, vegetables, nuts, seeds, legumes, whole grains, fish, and lean cuts of meat. Because a diet that emphasizes these items is not only nutritious but also satisfying and metabolically stimulating, the recipes have been developed with these fundamentals in mind. One of the things I like most about using intermittent fasting to manage my weight is that it does not intentionally limit any significant categories of foods, which is like a breath of fresh air.

When you manipulate the time and schedule of when you eat, you have more flexibility than dieting. This is due to the power of managing the timing and scheduling of when you eat. Instead of focusing on the beautiful foods that can be included in your diet, many diets tell you what foods you cannot consume.

In the following section, I will explain in greater detail why the foods you eat, and not the foods you avoid, will determine your success, not only during the next 21 days but also throughout what I hope will be a journey that lasts a lifetime and involves both healthy eating and intermittent fasting.

CALORIES, FULLNESS, AND FASTING

Consuming meals that are delectable and sufficient to meet one's nutritional needs is essential to success with the intermittent fasting method.

The metabolic benefits of fasting, the reduction in overall food consumption and calories that come with a shorter eating window, and the effects of higher protein intake are relied on by most beginner-friendly styles of intermittent fasting. One of the primary advantages of intermittent fasting is that, for the most part, you do not have to pay as close attention to the number of calories that you consume. Instead of counting calories, fasting depends on a reduced window of time during which you may consume food, enough consumption of protein, and a little increase in metabolic rate to facilitate weight reduction.

Some exceptions to this rule include instructing you to maintain your intake within a set range when participating in a weekly fast. I also understand that you may want some direction on calorie suggestions to assist your efforts to lose weight, and I am here to help. Although the precise calorie needs to promote weight reduction vary greatly from person to person based on age, gender, and activity level, I will try to make things as easy as possible for you to understand.

A daily calorie intake of 1,750 to 2,250 calories is recommended to facilitate healthy weight loss for most men.

Men over the age of 50 who engage in less physical activity will fall toward the lower end of that range, whereas younger men who are more active will be closer to the upper end of that range. A calorie range of 1,250 to 1,750 calories per day is recommended for most women to facilitate healthy weight reduction.

Women over the age of 50 who engage in less physical activity will fall toward the lower end of that range, whereas younger women who are more active will be closer to the upper end of that range. For comparison, the recommended calorie levels for men fasting solely for lifestyle and general health benefits rather than for weight loss are closer to 2,250 to 2,750 calories per day.

In comparison, the recommended calorie levels for women are closer to 1,750 to 2,250 calories per day.

In combination with the meal plans offered, those who are inclined to do so may utilize these values to manage their overall eating habits. It is essential to keep in mind that the meal plans provide you with a guide, but that the total number of calories will differ slightly depending on the day, the type of fast you choose, and the amount of each recipe you choose to consume.

Keeping this in mind will make it easier for you to adhere to the fast. In most instances, consuming simply one portion of each of the provided recipes will not give sufficient quantities of calories for the day.

This will allow you to add snacks or raise the recommended portion size of the meal you are preparing as you see appropriate.

You are more than welcome to double the serving sizes or even cut them in half, depending on the number of calories you need to consume each day and whether or not you intend to replace a lunch recommendation with dinner leftovers.

Take a moment with me while I elaborate on the significance of the nutrient known as protein. However, multiple studies have shown additional metabolic benefits when protein intake is increased by at least 50 percent, closer to 1.2 g/kg per day, and even up to 1.6 g/kg and beyond.

The recommended daily allowance for protein intake is 0.8 g/kg (grams per kilogram). Still, these studies have shown additional metabolic benefits when increasing protein intake by at least 50 percent. This is particularly true for people who participate in resistance training consistently.

At this level of protein intake, satiety tends to be greater, and the potential for weight loss is higher. This is at least partially due to what is known as the thermic effect of food, which means that it takes more energy for your body to break down protein than it does either carbohydrates or fat.

If you want to lose weight, increase your protein intake to this level. According to research published in the journal Obesity Facts in 2017, people who consumed the same amount of calories but a higher proportion of protein (1.34 g/kg per day as opposed to 0.8 g/kg per day) had bigger reductions in their body weight.

When a person has a greater protein consumption, they have a better chance of keeping their muscle mass even as they are losing weight, which is a very crucial factor to take into mind for active individuals and sportspeople.

In light of these facts, the focus for individuals participating in the 12:12, 16:8, or even OMAD fasts will be on plain old-fashioned healthy food that includes a lot of protein and fiber.

In both the 5:2 and ADMF plans, you are only allowed between 500 and 800 calories each day. On these days of the more difficult fast, it will be vital to focus on consuming a significant amount of protein and fiber. Conventionally, when we think of foods rich in protein, we think of things like chicken, eggs, meat, and dairy products, but when we think of meals high in fiber, we think of things like fruits and vegetables. These specific foods are diamonds for fasting and healthy eating in general since they are strong in protein and fiber. It is quite unusual for a full item to be high in these nutrients.

The most well-known and underappreciated items in this category are legumes, including black beans, lentils, chickpeas, kidney beans, etc.

On top of that, the cost of these foods is quite reasonable. The astounding amount of fiber and protein found in just one cup of beans is 17.5 grams. There is no other meal that provides such an abundance of these nutrients and a wide variety of vitamins, minerals, and antioxidants, all in a single serving.

POSITIVE THINKING AND REACHING YOUR GOALS

How you think about issues concerning your health and diet may significantly impact the results you get, just as is the case with all aspects of these topics.

This is very important to keep in mind during fasting, particularly for those just starting with the practice. Keep in mind that you have chosen to experiment with fasting because you want to, not because you must do so.

Keeping this information in mind, how do you plan to approach the final portion of your short each day? Will you look at it positively by anticipating the level of pleasure you will derive from having your first meal of the day? This way of thinking helps one succeed at intermittent fasting, mainly the more challenging kinds.

Because we all enjoy eating, intermittent fasting is inherently reward-driven; however, the biggest mistake I see clients make is getting too caught up in the structure and not listening to their body's cues. This is the biggest mistake I see clients make.

For illustration's sake, let's say someone is doing an alternate-day 16:8 fast, and on one of their fasting days, they wake up starving. Should they continue to fast even now?

My response is an emphatic no. One may say the same thing about waking up on a non-fasting day feeling full to the point where it is uncomfortable. Why wouldn't you give fasting some thought? As a result of the fact that so many of us eat in a ritualistic manner at predetermined times each day, we frequently lose touch with the degree to which we are, in fact, hungry.

Remember that intermittent fasting is a dynamic and intuitive tool that requires practice to become proficient at it, just like any other skill. You will put yourself in a much better position to be successful if you focus on finding ways to enjoy the process rather than concentrating solely on the result.

PLANNING YOUR EXERCISE

This chapter will walk you through how to mix intermittent fasting with physical activity in a manner that is beneficial to you.

It will also introduce the activities that will be a part of the workout section of your 21-day schedule.

While you are fasting, you should exercise.

First, let's distinguish between working out when fasting and working out while fasting.

A straightforward definition of "working out while fasting" is the practice of integrating some regular physical exercise into one's daily routine while simultaneously participating in a fasting regimen of some kind. You could opt to always exercise after breaking your fast if you are following the 16:8 method of fasting, for instance.

The practice of participating in physical exercise while in a fasting condition, meaning that one has gone without eating for a prolonged time, meant "working out while fasting." Not everyone should engage in physical activity when they are fasting.

While some of my customers do it without a second thought, others can't even bear to entertain the idea.

That is entirely OK; the priority here is your ease. It is vitally crucial to choose a fasting and exercise schedule tailored to your specific needs, which may need some trial and error. The information included in the following paragraphs will guide you on the proper route.

ADJUSTING TO YOUR FASTING BODY

How you adapt to regular intermittent fasting is determined by various things, such as the length of time you have spent fasting in the past, the protocol you are adhering to, and the bigger picture of how your diet and exercise routine are now structured.

Personal tastes and the extent to which one is comfortable are also relevant factors. If this is your first time fasting, it may take time for your body to adjust.

Longer fasts or days of continuous fasting may, for some individuals, be less favorable to effective workouts when fasted; however, this does not have to be the case at all times.

It is not caused for alarm if, after observing a prolonged fast, you discover that you lack the energy to engage in strenuous physical activity; this is a natural reaction. Regardless of how you choose to approach this topic, the following advice should always be considered.

STAY HYDRATED

Whether or not you are fasting, maintaining a healthy level of water is essential to your ability to grow and function.

However, when your body becomes used to the fasting routine, it becomes even more critical to ensure that you get enough water. According to the guidelines established by the Institute of Medicine in 2005, the recommended amount of water consumption is around 2.7 liters (91 ounces) per day for women and 3.7 liters (125 ounces) per day for men.

One cup of water equals 250 milliliters or 8.5 fluid ounces.

This guideline extends to include the water contained inside all meals and drinks in a strict sense. I do not encourage drinking excessive water to stave off hunger while you are on a fast. While drinking adequate water and other fluids may have a modest part in keeping you satisfied throughout your fast, I do not recommend drinking excessive water. If you are already at this hunger level, it is time to break your fast. It is entirely acceptable to break a fast early or not fast at all on a day when your body does not agree with it. Fasting is not designed to be excruciating, and it is entirely appropriate to break a fast early.

CAFFEINE HELPS

Caffeine is one of the naturally occurring performance enhancers that has been the subject of most research.

It improves alertness, lessens feelings of exhaustion, and may provide you the boost for your pre-workout that you need during the early phases of the adaption process to fasting. However, even while drinking caffeinated drinks like coffee and tea might motivate you to take daily fluids, the success or failure of your intermittent fasting regimen is not going to be determined by how much caffeine you eat.

It is thus not necessary to worry about this if you are not a person who regularly consumes coffee.

TAKE WHAT YOU EAT VERY SERIOUSLY.

When you hear this coming from a nutritionist, it probably does not surprise you.

Still, it's essential to ensure you don't underestimate the benefits of maintaining a healthy, well-balanced diet when participating in any intermittent fasting program.

Consuming the appropriate amounts of fiber, protein, and other nutrients is essential not only for achieving a state of satiety but also for maximizing one's performance in physical activity.

EXPERIMENT WITH YOUR APPROACH

I believe that intermittent fasting is a talent, and skills need practice to become proficient in them. It's possible that you won't find the type of fasting or workout program that works best for you on your first effort, but you shouldn't let that stop you from trying.

For example, when compared to working out later on the same day, some individuals report that working out while fasting results in a significantly different sensation than working out later on the same day.

Since you won't know until you give it a go, let's take a deeper look at how you may gradually move toward developing a suitable routine for you and your lifestyle.

ESTABLISHING A ROUTINE

In the next chapter, you will choose the method of fasting that is most appropriate for you; in this part, you will be encouraged to consider how physical activity may be included in that method. Strength, stamina, and mobility are the three primary benefits of physical exercise.

You can improve your strength by doing resistance training, endurance through aerobic exercise, and mobility by doing things like yoga and stretching.

It is ultimately up to you to choose how these exercises fit into your program, but the ones presented in this chapter will most likely be of assistance in doing so.

A well-rounded workout routine takes into account all of the factors listed above. Suppose you planned to exercise seven days a week, for instance. You may allocate three of those days to strength training, three to endurance training, and at least one day to mobility, stretching, and healing, all of which might also be included in your workouts on the other days.

Ask yourself, "Am I willing to exercise on a day when I haven't eaten?" On days when they don't intend to put in a lot of effort physically, many of my clients choose to go without food since it caters to their preferences and makes them feel more comfortable.

This is particularly true for those who work out in the morning. That begs the following inquiry: Do I plan to work out first thing in the morning or later in the evening?

I don't anticipate or want you to alter the time of day that you work out since I find that most individuals have a set preference and degree of comfort associated with the time of day that they work out. It is recommended that you modify your lifestyle to accommodate fasting rather than vice versa.

As an illustration of this principle, let's utilize the 16:8 method of fasting, which is pretty widespread. Most folks choose to observe a fast from the evening till the morning, from what I've seen. In this scenario, a 16:8 fast would abstain from food between eight hours in the evening and noon. This provides the typical individual who works a 9 to 5 job with three alternative possibilities, each with certain constraints:

1. Your first exercise of the day.

If you choose this strategy, it is possible that it may make your hunger worse and that it will be more difficult for you to fast, although this is less of a problem for daily fasts that last for a modest amount of time.

2. Late-afternoon exercise.

Although you will undoubtedly appreciate breaking you're fast more than usual, this stage can be the most physically taxing since you have reached the maximum amount of time you have been fasting for.

3. Late-evening exercise.

This enables you to exercise while in a well-fed condition; however, it is not always practicable due to schedule restrictions.

It may require you to exercise with a more significant amount of food in your stomach than you would desire. It is also possible that it will disrupt everyday sleep habits. There are benefits and drawbacks associated with each strategy. It all boils down to personal taste, comfort, and safety when it comes down to it.

Exercises That Don't Feel Like Exercises

Try a new kind of exercise on days when you don't feel like doing your standard multimove program or going for a jog for thirty minutes.

Sports and activities such as soccer, basketball, tennis, swimming, rock climbing, jumping rope, and bicycling contribute to significant body fat loss.

Also, don't be too quick to underestimate how much energy your body expends performing more hard domestic duties like mowing the lawn, cutting wood, or shoveling snow. These are all activities that require a significant amount of physical effort. In addition to the exercise routines presented in this book, there are many at-home routines, ranging from yoga to martial arts, that will truly shake up how you think about being fit.

Exercising On If For Woman

The practice of intermittent fasting is likely to be quite successful for a large number of women. This is because they have particular periods in which they do an excellent job of eating, and during such times they make sure that the food they consume is packed with various nutrients. However, including some physical activity in your daily routine is essential to optimize your outcomes and lose excess fat.

Despite this, recent research by the Swedish Institute of Sport and Health Sciences shows that decreasing the total quantity of carbs consumed in one's diet enables the body to burn calories more effectively and enhances the potential for muscle building.

In this research, ten cyclists who competed at the highest levels participated in an hour-long interval workout.

They maintained an average of 64 percent of their maximum aerobic capacity.

Before making any changes to their diet or exercise routine, these individuals had low or average glycogen stores in their muscular tissue. Ten muscle biopsies were collected before training, and then another ten were taken around three hours after the session. The findings indicated that physical activity was able to boost mitochondrial biogenesis even when the glycogen stores in the body were exhausted. This is the process that will result in the development of new mitochondria inside the cell.

The findings of this research led the authors to conclude that physical activity combined with a diet low in glycogen may be beneficial in increasing oxidative muscle capacity.

Working out when your body is already in a fasting condition is beneficial for several reasons. One of which is that the body goes through specific processes that assist keep and protecting the muscles from losing themselves.

Therefore, if you are short on fuel for an exercise, which you would, of course, be while you are on an intermittent fast, your body will start breaking down some of the other tissues in your body, but it will not break down the active muscle that you are utilizing.

Keeping Your Muscles in Good Shape Through Exercise

Diet is responsible for around 80 percent of the health advantages of leading a healthy lifestyle, according to the consensus of many qualified specialists.

Exercising is responsible for the remainder. This indicates that if you want to reduce weight, you need to concentrate on consuming meals to help you achieve that goal.

However, it is crucial to keep in mind that a healthy diet and regular exercise are necessary components.

The researchers analyzed the information provided by 11 contestants on "The Biggest Loser." The subjects' resting metabolic rate, total energy expenditure, and total body fat were assessed three times each.

At the beginning of the program, they were measured after six weeks; after 30 weeks, they were measured again.

The researchers were able to quantify the effect of changes in food and exercise that resulted in weight reduction by using a human metabolic model. This allowed them to examine how both factors contributed to achieving the goal of losing weight.

The researchers discovered that diet alone was responsible for most of the weight decrease. However, around 65 percent of this weight loss was due to a reduction in body fat. Lean muscle mass was the primary contributor to the remaining weight loss in the body. Exercise on its own only led to a decrease in body fat and a minor increase in the amount of lean muscle mass.

Combining Physical Activity and Dietary Restriction

A few components need to come together for you to have a successful fitness program that includes both high-intensity training and intermittent fasting.

If you want to achieve this, you need to do a couple of things. If despite your preference, you find that you do not have the energy to continue with the exercises when you do this, then it is time for you to make some adjustments.

In most cases, shortening the duration of the fast from its original length will provide the desired results. It is expected that you would feel fantastic while participating in intermittent fasting; if this is not the case, it is time to reconsider your strategy. When working out in the occasional challenging setting, there are two primary considerations that you need to keep in mind.

The first one has to do with how you consume your meals. It's important to remember that calorie restriction is just one aspect of intermittent fasting.

You are not supposed to cheat yourself out of having excellent outcomes. Instead, all that is required is careful planning of meal times to prevent you from overeating for the better part of the day. You may get a brief opportunity to eat, perhaps later in the day or the evening. You will have fasted for 21 hours if you do not eat between the hours of 4 and 7 in the evening.

The majority of males can successfully abstain from food and drink for somewhere between 12 and 18 hours. People often choose to run for 16 hours since it is the shortest amount of time that can be squeezed into their hectic schedules. You will choose what meets your requirements the most effectively by ensuring that you take advantage of all the perks.

If you have problems staying entirely away from food throughout the day, you should limit your supper to a modest quantity of low-glycemic, sweet foods and keep the portion size very small. Eggs poached in water, whey protein, vegetables, fruit, and other nutritious alternatives, should be had every four to six hours. On the days when you decide to get some shut-eye, it is in your best interest to abstain from eating for at least three hours before going to bed.

Doing this will assist in decreasing the oxidative damage that is caused to your system, and it will also make it much simpler to accomplish intermittent fasting.

In addition, you should break your fasts with a recovery meal on the days when you engage in physical activity.

On days when you have to work out while fasting, you need to have a recovery meal around thirty minutes after you complete your workout. The improved muscle repair that includes whey protein in your diet is simple to integrate. After you have finished eating that meal, it is highly recommended that you go without food again until the time of your primary meal that evening. It is essential to consume a proper recovery meal after each training session that you complete.

This will guarantee that your body receives the necessary amount of energy and prevent any injury to your muscles or brain. Do not miss this meal, and after your exercise, have it within the next half an hour at the latest. If you believe it will be difficult to abstain from food for 12 to 18 hours, you may obtain the same benefits from exercise and fasting by missing breakfast and working out on an empty stomach first thing in the morning.

This will have the same outcomes as abstaining from food for 12 to 18 hours. This is because consuming a substantial meal before a workout, especially one that is high in carbohydrate content, suppresses the sympathetic nervous system, which in turn diminishes the benefits of your activity on your body's ability to burn fat.

Although most individuals have been instructed to consume a large number of carbohydrates before exercising to increase their endurance and see results, this strategy is counterproductive to the objectives that you have set for yourself. Consuming excessive carbohydrates activates the parasympathetic nervous system, which encourages the body to store calories and carbohydrates for later use as a source of energy. If you are running and doing the problematic irregular, this is probably the last thing you anticipate. Therefore it will be easy to notice more significant results in a shorter amount of time.

Some Suggestions to Help You Get the Most Out of Your Workouts

The exercises on an irregular calendar are not intended to be particularly challenging. However, you may expect to feel better overall, gain muscle, and lose weight if you exercise regularly and get lots of physical activity. When you are training on an irregular fast, some of the things you can do to ensure that you are progressing very well are as follows:

1. If you've never finished a weightlifting program before, you'll need to take things carefully at first to avoid injuring yourself. Even if you're getting back into your regular workout routine, it's essential to recognize the progress you've made and gradually

work up to your previous level of intensity to gauge how the changes will impact your overall performance.

2. When you reach a point where you feel comfortable, add more weight; once you reach a point where you feel comfortable, you must continue to add more weight. After some time, the weights that you continue to train with will start to seem relatively light, and if you don't make any adjustments to your routine, you'll notice that your performance is decreasing. This does not imply that you should push your body beyond its capabilities. Still, it indicates that if you want to see sustained success, you should strive to make your workout regimen progressively more

challenging regularly. When it comes to building lean muscle, more repetitions with a more significant weight are preferable. However, if you are interested in lean muscle creation, you should attempt doing fewer repetitions with greater weight. This allows for a more effective draining of the body, which will result in improved results.

3. It is important to remember to warm up and cool down after your workout. Just because you need to modify your eating routines does not permit you to skip your exercise routine's warm-up and cool-down phases. It will take at least five minutes to stretch the muscles at the beginning and conclusion of an exercise session to

increase performance. Still, it will also lessen the probability of an injury occurring.

4. Maintain your fitness level; when we go to the gym, we tend to be too preoccupied with seeing how much weight we can lift at a given moment. On the other hand, form is really of more significance than content. Therefore, it is better not to worry.

The following are some of the social and life benefits of intermittent fasting:

+ When you stop worrying so much about needing to deviate from your routine to eat continuously, you will be amazed to discover how much more time you have available to devote to other pursuits. You will have more time to devote to other activities without being distracted by your hunger pangs when you engage in intermittent fasting. It helps you save money because when you don't have to spend money on meals in a state of fear, you typically spend less overall. You could be taking in the same number of calories, but if you focus on just one meal each day, you'll have more money in your pocket.

It makes traveling simpler since you won't have to stress about the dietary decisions you have to make when you visit other nations because of this. This offers you more space and prevents you from gaining fat, and promotes the partitioning of nutrients in your body. Your stamina is much boosted as a result of this because intermittent fasting relies exclusively on the infinite fatty acids stored in the body; as a result, your stamina is significantly increased. As soon as your body has adjusted to the fasting, you won't have to worry about your energy supply running out.

+ Admiration: Not everyone may approve of your actions, but I can assure you that your extraordinary capacity for self-control will impress many members of your family and friends. This boosts confidence and makes you feel excellent about yourself.

+ Your willpower will improve as a result since intermittent fasting doesn't take a lot of it from you because it's so simple to execute. Maintaining your resolve will provide you with a sense of self-control and achievement. According to research, increasing your willpower in one sector of your life by gaining control and succeeding can enhance your willpower in other areas of your life.

- It helps prevent ego depletion because, while you are practicing intermittent fasting, you tend to make fewer choices about food during the day. This, in turn, protects you from weariness and ego depletion. However, according to research, decision-making depletes your energy reserves, which in turn lowers your capacity to make sound decisions.

- You will have more clarity when distinguishing between a false appetite and true hunger if you participate in intermittent fasting. This kind of fasting allows you to comprehend the distinction between the two better. Furthermore, this allows you to realize the difference between what you need and what you desire, which is an innovative and powerful concept.

+ It helps you get over the dread of becoming hungry: Your voracious hunger will become easier to manage as you practice intermittent fasting. The longer you go without food, the less hungry you are likely to feel. This will enable you to quit planning when you will consume meals or snacks in the future.

+ It enables you to enjoy meals without feeling any sense of obligation or limitation:

The practice of intermittent fasting is an effective method for losing weight without the accompanying feelings of deprivation or guilt. You can consume food without experiencing guilt when engaging in intermittent fasting, which helps you burn fat even in hard-to-target regions.

WHAT TO EAT AND WHAT NOT TO EAT

Regardless of the strategy you choose to use when it comes to an intermittent fast, you must have a grasp of the types of foods that are beneficial to consume and those that should be avoided throughout your efforts. You will need to know precisely what you should consume on the days when you are supposed to be fasting unless you are planning on going without any solid meals for a whole day. In the same vein, it might be beneficial for you to have an idea of what would work best for you on days when you are not fasting because keep in mind that the fact that you could be on one of your non-fast days does not indicate that it would be a good idea for you to travel to the city and overindulge at a buffet where you can eat as much as you like.

What to Consume

Coffee

Even though it is not technically a meal, coffee is a perfect addition to any fast day since it has no calories and may be enjoyed as a beverage. The vast majority of us need a cup of coffee first thing in the morning.

Therefore this is unquestionably excellent news for those of us who take pleasure in our Joe first thing in the morning. In addition, coffee can help alleviate some of the uncomfortable side effects of fasting. If, for example, the first few hours of your fast leave you feeling a little tired and drained of energy, you may find that a robust and flavorful cup of coffee helps alleviate these side effects.

However, remember that the coffee must be consumed immediately after being removed from the pot, without adding any sugar or cream to it.

The flavor of black coffee without any added sugar may take some of you a little while to get used to, but in the long term, you'll be much better off if you give up the sugar and cream.

Raspberries

Raspberries are a low-calorie snack that won't ruin your fast day and, at the same time, will help you maintain regular bowel movements by providing you with a healthy dosage of fiber.

Raspberries are available year-round. Raspberries are an excellent source of beneficial vitamins and minerals and the inflammation-fighting antioxidants found in abundance in these berries. This is beneficial for protecting against arthritis as well as other degenerative disorders. It has even been suggested that raspberries help protect against cancer in some circumstances.

This is because "Ellagic acid," a potent cancer-fighting phytochemical, may be abundant in the plant. If you are on a fast day and have nothing else to eat, a bowl of plain, unsweetened raspberries would be an excellent decision to make for your diet.

Beans and other legumes are low in calories.

Beans, beans, the fruit of all enchantment. The more food you consume, the more fat you will be able to burn throughout your fast. Beans and other legumes, in general, have a low-calorie count and are filled with a variety of beneficial elements.

They also include a substantial amount of protein, which helps to ensure that your muscles continue to get fuel even after your body's fat reserves are exhausted.

Despite their small size, beans, and other legumes pack a powerful punch when it comes to their ability to promote weight loss when consumed during intermittent fasting. Peas, black beans, lentils, and garbanzo beans are some of the legumes that do the best when it comes to the practice of intermittent fasting.

Blueberries

These delicious fruity snacks are not only low in calories but also rich in antioxidants, which helps to guarantee that the body is kept free of harmful free radicals that, over time, might ruin the tissue in the body.

While fasting, eating blueberries, which are known to strengthen the immune system, is a fantastic way to ensure that you do not get ill or otherwise weakened. Flavonoids are found in blueberries, and if you eat them regularly over an extended period, they have the potential to lower your body mass index (BMI) overall.

This is another one of the cool things about blueberries (Body Mass Index). This is unquestionably a fortunate turn of events. And I forgot to say... They have a wonderful flavor as well!

Eggs

Eggs may be prepared in various ways, including hard boiling, scrambling, or poaching, but regardless of how you prepare them, they are an excellent source of nutrients with a low-calorie count. Eggs simply appear to be particularly well-suited for this endeavor.

Eggs contain a significant quantity of proteins and tend to remain in your stomach for a prolonged period, which leaves you feeling full and content.

On the day that you are fasting, if you are giving yourself a small allocation of fewer than 500 calories, including a couple of eggs in your meal is not going to break your fast.

Breast meat from lean chicken

A plate of lean chicken breast is an excellent way to conclude a short day that shouldn't exceed your allocation of 500 calories, provided that you are not engaging in a fast that lasts for 24 hours. The lean chicken breast is an excellent source of protein and does not include the same amount of fat or filler as other cuts of meat.

It is also an essential ingredient that may be used in various recipes and meals.

You will discover many recipes in this book for one that makes the most of the benefits that may be gained from consuming a piece of lean chicken. In light of those above, you should prioritize storing up some lean chicken breast to be well prepared for your subsequent intermittent fast.

Fish

On a day when you are restricting your caloric intake, fish, like chicken, may provide you with a sufficient amount of protein without exceeding your daily calorie limit.

Omega-3 fatty acids may be found in abundance in fish due to the fish's high omega-3 content. But don't let the term "fat" put you off since omega-3 fatty acids are beneficial to your body.

There is a rationale that every health food shop has omega-3 pills in many aisles. Because omega-3 fatty acids have been shown to protect our hearts, significantly lower blood pressure, remove plaque from arteries, and even stave off heart attacks and strokes.

Fish is sometimes referred to as a "brain food" because of its capacity to assist in the enhancement of cognitive function. Fish is undeniably tasty, yet it also provides many health benefits. Make sure you put it to good use.

Veggies

One need not adhere to a vegetarian diet to recognize the significant contribution that vegetables may make to one's health. On the day that you do not observe the fast and every day in between, vegetables may act as a stabilizing influence.

Vegetables provide us with lots of essential nutrients, but they also give us a healthy dosage of fiber, which assists in maintaining regular bowel movements.

Because of their generally low-calorie content, vegetables are pretty versatile when it comes to meal preparation and may be combined with a wide variety of dishes. Make sure that you have a good supply of fresh vegetables available.

Unprocessed Grains

Whole grains are an excellent source of nourishment, regardless of whether one is fasting or not on a given day. These morsels will not cause you to break your fast and will yet leave you feeling full and pleased.

This is in contrast to refined grains, which cause an increase in insulin levels. This cookbook has quite a few recipes, most of which call for the usage of whole grains. If you are ever unsure, the safest bet is to opt for whole grains to replace bread. This makes for a beautiful substitute for bread.

Yogurt

People usually think of yogurt as one of the first healthy foods that spring to mind when they think of meals that are good for them. Even when you are fasting, eating yogurt may boost your metabolism and provide you with more energy. Yogurt is a fantastic source of nutrients.

Yogurts often include a healthy serving of probiotic bacteria, which, once consumed, continue their beneficial effects on the digestive tract even after the yogurt has been consumed. The so-called "good gut bacteria" are being emphasized more and more as the critical factor in maintaining overall health by medical professionals.

Yogurt is a risk-free method of consuming a significant amount of it. When it comes to being ready for your intermittent fasting routine, yogurt is one food that may most definitely be of assistance to you.

Chocolate with a dark hue

I know that not everyone likes dark chocolate; maybe one has to develop a taste for it over time. However, the positive effects on your health may be seen right away, regardless of whether or not it takes you some time to understand it fully.

The consumption of dark chocolate may provide you with a boost in energy while also reinforcing your body with beneficial antioxidants. Antioxidants of the kind that are capable, among other things, of warding off cancer.

To put it more simply, dark chocolate is a potent substance. When it comes to intermittent fasting, one of the best foods to consume is dark chocolate since it has so many advantages.

Coconut Oil

Coconut oil is a proven metabolism booster that has a low-calorie count. Consuming it throughout your intermittent fasting time will help get your system up and running again.

Coconut oil is beneficial because it does not stimulate the creation of insulin in the body, unlike other oils.

You don't have to worry about breaking your fast if you use coconut oil in any capacity, whether as a supplement or a helper in the kitchen. It's quite a lovely addition to any dish.

What You Should Not Consume

Soda

What, no soda? You've got to be kidding me! I'm sorry, guys, but unfortunately, it's too true. A refreshing fountain drink of soda is one of my guilty pleasures as much as the next person.

You will not be able to participate in intermittent fasting if you continue to drink soda since it breaks the fasting cycle. This is not intended as a kind of punishment; instead, it is just the nature of the beast.

After all, avoiding sugar is one of the most critical aspects of an intermittent fast and should be one of your primary goals. While we are fasting, we do not drink sugary sodas to give our metabolism something to chew on. This is done so that our bodies will begin burning fat deposits that are already there. As a result, if you want to keep up with your habit of engaging in intermittent fasting, you will need to avoid drinking soda for the time being.

Heavily Processed food

The use of processed foods is discouraged, which you have probably already understood from reading this book.

Anything that has been processed and packaged will have a ton of preservatives put into it, which, although typically innocuous, will have a long-term impact on your system over time. Anything that has been processed and packaged will have a ton of preservatives packed into it. Consuming foods that have been heavily processed will also have a direct negative impact on your metabolism. When it comes to intermittent fasting, the ideal option is to consume as fresh as possible food.

Sugary Sweets

The consumption of sugary sweets during an intermittent fast would be entirely unhelpful, in the same way, that drinking sugary drinks would be.

After all, an intermittent fast aims to train the body to burn stored fat rather than sugar and carbohydrates as its primary fuel source to reduce overall body fat percentage. Consuming sugary sweets would prevent this process and would instead add additional trash to the fat already stored in our trunks. Therefore, when you are engaging in intermittent fasting, you absolutely should not consume any sugary or sweet foods at any cost.

Alcohol

Let me start by saying that I don't intend to ruin the fun in any way, shape, or form, but let me just go ahead and say it. Consuming alcohol while on an intermittent fast is not recommended.

What is the cause? Consuming alcohol has a direct bearing on how efficiently the metabolism burns fat. And the last thing you want to do is screw with your fat-burning metabolism in the middle of your fast since that would be a disaster for your diet! In addition, alcohol contains carbohydrates, sugars, other similar substances, and calories. Therefore, much like drinking and driving, the combination of fasting and drinking should be avoided.

The Processed Grains

On the other hand, refined grains will have a markedly detrimental effect on your fast, in contrast to whole grains.

After being digested, refined grains will change into sugar in their place. The goal of intermittent fasting is to train your body to burn fat rather than sugar for fuel.

This is accomplished by alternating periods of eating customarily spaced out by periods of fasting. Consuming refined grains, which are eventually converted into sugar, thus, entirely nullifies this process. Additionally, it will cause an increase in your insulin levels. Processed grains should be avoided at all costs if there is any way to do so.

Trans-Fat

As simply as possible, trans fats are awful for you. They are not a source of any benefit. And most importantly, there is absolutely no way that consuming them can help your fast in any way. Therefore, during the time that you are engaging in an intermittent fast, you should refrain from consuming any foods that contain trans fat, which includes some types of milk and meat products.

It causes an increase in cholesterol and insulin levels, and it destroys any possibility that you may have had of having a successful fast.

Fast Food

Even though we call it "fast food," the burgers and fries that we bag from restaurants like McDonald's are not exactly the healthiest thing to consume while you are doing an intermittent fast, if you take a glance at the highly processed, carb-heavy meal that McDonald's serves, then you'll probably be able to grasp my point.

Precautions and Mistakes

Cautionary Measures to Take While Traveling On If

It is a shift in lifestyle that has to be included in your regular activities daily.

Altering our food patterns might have a significant impact on our day-to-day lives since our eating habits are an essential component of our lives. As a result, making a rash decision to alter anything is not recommended. Instead, you will need to make some adjustments to your diet and gradually extend the window of time during which you are fasting.

In the following section, we will talk about the many preventative measures that may be taken to ensure a seamless transition:

Put extra effort into watching what you eat. Remaining hungry for a long is not an easy challenge. It is not only a question of exercising self-control, but it also has a significant influence on the functioning of your physiological systems. It is essential for you to have a nutritious diet that may keep your body functioning normally even when you are not consuming any food. Your body stores a lot of fat, which may be broken down and utilized as an energy source. Nevertheless, your body will need training in order to begin the fat-burning process. The majority of the carbohydrates we consume come from the food that we eat on a daily basis. It indicates that glucose is being used as fuel for the body. The body is pushed to burn fat as fuel when someone does intermittent fasting.

You may be of assistance to the cause by reducing the number of carbs in the meals you eat and increasing the amounts of fat and protein that you take in. Maintaining a ketogenic diet will bring you a significant amount of success along this route. You must ensure that the carbohydrates you eat are not simple carbs. Because of this, you should stay away from refined flours as well as bread, biscuits, crackers, bagels, soda, and anything else that includes refined sugar. These substances are exceptionally quickly absorbed and cause urges for other food to be consumed. They will make it challenging for you to maintain your fasts. It would help if you ate a lot of green leafy vegetables because, in addition to providing vitamins and minerals, they are also an excellent source of dietary fiber. You should only consume foods made with whole grains since these foods include a high level of healthy fiber. They take a while to digest, so they keep you feeling full for a more extended period of time.

If you are currently dealing with a health issue that necessitates you to eat regularly or if your energy requirements are high as a result of something like pregnancy, you should not make a move to intermittent fasting. Before commencing a regimen of intermittent fasting, you should always see your primary care physician. Because it is such a significant shift in one's way of life, all appropriate safety measures should be taken before making the transition.

Always be sure to take into account the elements that are impacting your way of life. It will be difficult for you to get your mind off of food while you are fasting if you work in a restaurant or another environment in which there is always food around. A longer eating window allows you to keep up with the 14:10 fasting schedule without any difficulty. It would be impossible to stick to a fasting schedule like 20:4 or alternate days if you did that. Your thoughts will never stop being preoccupied with food, and as a result, life will become more difficult for you. As a result, you will also need to choose an appropriate fasting strategy.

Never think of the fasting period as a kind of self-inflicted punishment at that time. A lot of individuals continue to eat during the fasting window because they believe that going without food for an extended period of time would be exceedingly tricky. They would undoubtedly have an adamant time with the fast. Your eating windows need to be as normal and balanced as possible for the best results. It is not necessary for you to overeat since doing so will just make it more difficult for you to fast.

Get rid of any unhealthy food products or processed foods that you have in your house. Having a healthy lifestyle should be a habit; it is not something that just happens by happenstance. If you want to maintain a healthy weight and live a healthy lifestyle, you need to eliminate the temptations to consume unhealthy foods, and the first place you should focus on doing this is in your refrigerator. Take out the goods that contain a lot of sugar or foods that have been processed. Get in the habit of eating well, and it will become second nature to you.

Get rid of soda and any other drinks that only add extra calories to your body without providing any nutritional value. Take care of your fitness program without any difficulty. If you've been performing high-intensity activities or strength training, you should continue doing them on the days when you aren't restricting your food intake. It is imperative that you give your body the opportunity to relax during the fasting days, at the very least in the beginning stages of the shift. As you get more used to the regimen, you will be able to ramp up the intensity of the workouts you do.

On days when you are expected to fast, you may participate in activities such as yoga, cardiovascular workouts, walking, or running.

As you reduce the number of foods you consume and the number of times you consume them, you increase your risk of developing a vitamin and mineral shortage.

You can find that taking certain supplements of essential minerals and vitamins helps you deal with this problem. Some of the supplements that may be of assistance to you during this time of change are potassium, magnesium, and the B vitamin complex.

It cannot be emphasized enough that you should drink a lot of water throughout the day. When you fast, your body goes through a number of different detoxification processes, which is something you really need to be aware of.

It causes a significant amount of detoxification, and as a result, your body will begin to shed a lot of water.

If you are not getting enough water in your diet, you will experience symptoms of dehydration. This is potentially risky beyond a certain point. Therefore, it is imperative that you consume a lot of water.

Your body loses a lot of minerals in addition to water, which is why you should add a pinch of sea salt to some water or take some electrolytes.

Both of these options are available to you. Because of this, you won't experience any of the symptoms associated with dehydration, like feeling weary or having other issues.

Reduce the amount of alcohol and cigarettes you smoke.

This is a standard piece of advice that can be used in any circumstance; however, it is particularly crucial when you are following the intermittent fasting method since alcohol contains a lot of sugar, which causes your insulin levels to increase and also causes damage to your liver.

Because smoking causes a significant amount of harm to your health, you should make every effort to cut down on your cigarette use if you discover that you are unable to quit the habit entirely.

If you suffer any of the following symptoms while you are fasting, and they remain after you break your fast, you must immediately stop the fasting and make an appointment with a doctor.

These symptoms may be brought on by a number of different conditions; however, only a medical professional can provide accurate diagnosis and recommendations for treatment moving forward. Due to the fact that the female hormonal system is rather sensitive, it is essential to seek the guidance of a medical professional at all times. Some of the red flags that you should keep an eye out for are:

Even When I Have Nothing in My Stomach, I Have to Throw Up

There are a number of potential causes of vomiting, including inflammation of the stomach lining, an electrolyte imbalance, or even something more serious going on in your stomach; as a result, you should see a medical professional if the issue continues.

Feeling Like Fire Is Coming From Your Stomach

Gastritis is another potential source of this condition; nevertheless, if it continues despite your best efforts, you should seek medical attention since there are likely other factors at play here.

Continued episodes of diarrhea

There are a number of potential causes for loose stools, but if they are not stopped in a timely manner, they may lead to dehydration, weakness, and a wide variety of other health issues.

You really must get medical attention right now.

Fainting

Practitioners of intermittent fasting may experience feelings of lightheadedness, dizziness, and weakness.

These sensations are common side effects of the transformation your body is through, and they will go away very quickly. These symptoms may also manifest themselves as sugar withdrawal symptoms in certain people.

If you experience fainting more than once in a short period of time, you should get in touch with a medical professional as soon as possible since this is not something that should be seen as a typical occurrence.

An ache in the Stomach or the Chest

You may have these symptoms sometimes for a variety of causes; however, if they continue beyond a short period of time, you should make an appointment with your primary care physician.

Erratic Periods

If you have started altogether skipping your periods after beginning intermittent fasting, if the amount of bleeding that occurs during your periods has significantly increased, or if you are getting blood spots even when they shouldn't be, you should make an appointment with your primary care physician as soon as possible.

Common Mistakes

You have probably already heard about the advantages of intermittent fasting, which are what have contributed to the rise in popularity of this eating pattern.

If you've chosen to give this way of eating a go but haven't seen any changes in your body yet, it's possible that you're not following the instructions properly. It is possible for you to accidentally commit a number of errors that will make the experience more challenging for you.

To ensure that your trip with intermittent fasting is fruitful, it is imperative that you steer clear of the following frequent errors:

Making Significant Alterations to Your Daily Routine

It might be challenging to make the transition from eating every three to four hours to eating within an eight-hour span all at once. This is due to the fact that you are likely to have constant feelings of hunger.

This may cause one to feel discouraged. In point of fact, this is the moment at which some individuals decide to give up on their effort at intermittent fasting, long before their bodies have really had a chance to acclimate to the change from their typical eating habits.

In general, it might take up to ten days before you can settle into your new eating pattern and cease feeling hungry during the fasting window. This is because your body needs time to adjust to the changes.

Start by increasing the number of hours that pass between meals until you are able to reach a period of fasting that lasts for 12 hours without feeling uncomfortable. This will help you make the shift more easily. You may then build on this to get to a point where you are fasting for at least 16 hours and eating for just 8 hours.

Putting Your Faith in God and Your Fasting Before Him

When you first begin practicing intermittent fasting, it is probable that your mind and thoughts will begin to revolve around the practice itself. Because you are restricting your food intake, you could discover that you are avoiding social situations like going to supper with your family or declining invitations to gatherings.

Because of this, it is often impossible to maintain intermittent fasting over time, and it also makes it less pleasurable.

Instead, you should think about putting up a timetable for intermittent fasting that is compatible with your lifestyle and schedule so that you can easily handle the social engagements that you have planned.

After all, intermittent fasting is not a diet in the traditional sense since it does not dictate what foods you should consume.

Consuming Excess Calories During Your Allotted Eating Time

After you first start fasting, it might be tempting to overeat when the fasting period is done. It's possible that this was triggered when you tried to excuse your behavior by telling yourself that you needed to make up for missed calories or that you were just starving. This is not an intelligent strategy, mainly if your goal in fasting is to reduce your body fat percentage and obtain a healthier weight.

In addition, consuming an excessive amount of food after having fasted for a lengthy period of time may lead to a variety of health issues, including abdominal pain and diarrhea, amongst others.

As a result, it is in your best interest to have a meal plan that you can use as a reference in order to be ready to cook a nutritious meal when the time comes for you to break your fast. Make it a priority to use whole foods wherever it is feasible, such as an abundance of veggies, lean protein, and whole grains.

Having Given Up Way Too Soon

The pattern of eating known as intermittent fasting may seem to be straightforward on paper, but in practice, it may be challenging to adhere to. This pattern of eating naturally reduces the number of calories you consume by reducing the amount of time you spend between meals.

As a result, you are able to function on a lower calorie intake. This indicates that not every strategy will be suitable for you since it depends on how you live your life.

As a result, rather than giving up, you should practice patience or attempt a new way of fasting other than the one you began with until you discover one that is suitable for you.

Insufficient Physical Activity or Exercise

Before heading to the gym, a pre-workout snack is something that many people do.

As a result, the idea of exercising while you're fasting could seem completely strange to you. If you are thinking along these lines, it is crucial to keep in mind that your body will always have ample energy, which it stores as fat in order to utilize when you haven't eaten for a decent amount of time when you don't feed yourself.

Even in this case, you should always be sure to check with your primary care physician before engaging in physical activity while you are fasting.

In any other case, you may stick to your regular exercise plan, or you might even experiment with some low-impact activities like walking.

If you are going to exercise the following day after going without food for the previous 24 hours, it is essential to have a meal that is high in protein so that you may speed up the pace at which your muscles will grow.

Drinking Wrong Liquids

When you are fasting, it is essential to ensure that you drink enough water so that you do not have feelings of weakness or extreme hunger.

During the course of the day, you are welcome to consume water, tea, or coffee. However, neither tea nor coffee should have any sugar added to them.

Because they have the potential to alter your insulin levels and may put a stop to the process of autophagy, which is something you want to encourage, it is essential to steer clear of any drinks and beverages that have a high amount of calories or protein.

This indicates that you should steer clear of diet sodas as well as anything else that has a significant amount of added sugar.

It is essential to keep in mind that certain zero-calorie sweeteners may still have an influence on your insulin levels and may cause you to feel more hungry.

You may utilize applications that help you monitor your hydration if you are having trouble drinking enough during the day. This will ensure that you stay hydrated by drinking beverages such as water, coffee, and tea throughout the day.

Consuming Foods That Are Bad For You

Although the primary emphasis of intermittent fasting is on when you eat rather than the quality of the food you consume, you should still make an effort to consume nutritious meals, mainly if your goal is to reduce your body fat percentage.

You will have a difficult time reaching your health objective, for example, if the majority of the meals you consume are processed foods, and you overlook the importance of eating whole foods, which are components of a diet that is nutritionally sound.

As you get used to your new eating pattern, you should make an effort to gradually adapt your diet such that it includes selections that are healthy for you. Because of this, you won't have to attempt to completely revamp everything all at once, which will make your strategy more sustainable.

Making the Wrong Choice for How to Do Intermittent Fasting

You have to make things as easy as possible for yourself if you want to be successful, and one way to do so is to choose an intermittent fasting protocol that is compatible with your lifestyle and the objectives you want to accomplish.

If you choose an intermittent fasting strategy that is incompatible with your lifestyle, you are setting yourself up for failure even before you begin the program. When you fast, it is crucial to keep in mind that critical elements of your life, such as your employment, your social life, and your health objectives, are likely to be impacted.

Consuming Insufficient Calories During Your Allotted Fasting Period

When you have an overly ambitious weight reduction goal, you may find that you are tempted to eat too little within your eating window, despite the fact that you are fasting for extended periods of time.

This is counterintuitive since there is a possibility that not eating enough food may lead to an increase in weight. Here's why: when you consume too little, your body begins to break down and cannibalize its own muscular mass, which essentially slows down your metabolism.

Your capacity to keep the same amount of fat or shed fat in the future may be hindered if you do not have a suitable amount of metabolic muscle mass.

This is made much worse by the fact that intermittent fasting is based on arbitrary temporary rules rather than the actual indications from the body. This makes the situation even more difficult.

You're Placing An Excessive Amount Of Emphasis On When You Eat While Ignoring The Importance Of What You Consume.

The primary distinction between intermittent fasting and several other diets is that the former focuses primarily on the passage of time while the latter is mute on the subject of what foods to consume. As a result of this, it is simple to get caught up in the trap of eating meals that are unhealthy, which will result in you nullifying the advantages of fasting.

Milkshakes and beer are two examples of beverages and foods that can undoubtedly slow down your progress, mainly if they are drunk in excess and without moderation. Keep in mind that fasting is not magic since the advantages it provides are dependent on the fact that you get to lower the number of calories you ingest just by cutting down on the amount of time you spend eating.

Carrying out an excessive number of activities at the same time

If you have made a number of choices with the intention of making significant changes to your way of life, you should make every effort to avoid making all of those changes at once. For instance, you shouldn't make drastic dietary changes, overdo your workouts, and fast all at the same time.

This is the same as taking in more than you are capable of chewing. Therefore, you should make the modifications gradually so that you don't start off by engaging in daily exercise, fasting for a lengthy period of time, and cutting down on calories all at the same time.

Because your body is able to flourish with a bit of stress, but too much stress is not healthy for it, this can only lead to issues. At the same time, your body is able to thrive under a bit of stress.

Obsessing Over Timings

One of the benefits of practicing intermittent fasting is that it trains your body to respond more appropriately to actual bouts of hunger.

This is because the majority of the time, what we think is hungry is really thirst creeping up on us. Not every four hours, but much more often between 16 to 24 hours, true hunger will strike. Instead of planning when you will eat or eat at random intervals throughout the day, you need to listen to your body to determine the times at which you ought to take in food. If you continue to count the hours until you can eat, your body will not grasp the real hunger signals that it is sending out.

Are You Experiencing Guilt Because You Ate Outside of Your Allotted Feeding Window?

When it comes to intermittent fasting, one of the most significant things that most people overlook is how crucial it is to pay attention to your body, particularly in the beginning when you're just getting started.

 If you are unable to continue a fast because you are feeling too hungry, it is OK to break your fast and consume some food.

If you disregard the signs that your body is giving you that it's hungry, you run the risk of developing an unhealthy connection with food, which may lead to feelings of guilt if you have to eat outside of your standard feeding window. This puts you at risk of developing an eating problem in the long run, which is why it's risky.

In order for you to experience success with intermittent fasting, you need to ensure that you are carrying out the practice in the correct manner.

This requires a number of steps, including finding the appropriate plan, maintaining the appropriate level of motivation, and paying attention to your body's needs. The essential thing you can do is pay attention to your routines and make sure that the routines you engage in are solely healthy routines.

You shouldn't simply start intermittent fasting because everyone else is doing it; you should start it because you are serious about changing your lifestyle. It is in your best interest to conduct as much study as possible on this pattern of eating before beginning the shift into it. This will ensure that you are as well-informed as possible during the process.

YOUR 21-DAY PLAN

BE PREPARED TO BRING YOUR 21-DAY PLAN TO LIFE; it will play a vital part in getting you started on the road to success with intermittent fasting. However, it is not an either/or proposition. Every week is different and particularly tailored to one of the six different types of fasting that are covered in the book. If you begin the program with a kind of fast that does not work for you during the first week, you are free to switch to a different type of fast throughout the second and third weeks of the program.

Essentials for the Cabinets, the Fridge, and the Freezer Before we get started with week one and all the awesome things that come with it, I'm going to go over some nutritional fundamentals that will play a significant part in the next 21 days that you have ahead of you.

You will need to have these pantry essentials in order to create any of the recipes in the book, but it is not necessary to purchase everything at once. Before you construct your grocery list for each week, you should first evaluate how many people, in addition to yourself, you will be cooking for, how many leftovers you may have (if any), and how many calories you need to consume in order to fulfill the requirements of your chosen fast. Remember that if you have leftovers from one meal, you may store them in the refrigerator or freezer and then use them to substitute for another meal on the plan. You can do this as long as you remember to do so.

PANTRY ESSENTIALS

Healthy Fats

- ✓ Avocado

- ✓ Butter

- ✓ Coconut

- ✓ Coconut oil

- ✓ Nuts and nut butter: almonds, cashews, peanuts, pecans, pistachios, walnuts, and so on

- ✓ Olive oil

- ✓ Olives

- ✓ Seeds: chia, flax, hemp, pepita, pumpkin, sesame, sunflower, and so on

- ✓ Sesame oil

- ✓ Tahini

- ✓ Tahini sauce

- ✓ Tahini sauce

- ✓ Tahini sauce

- ✓ Tahini

Beans and other legumes include black beans, chickpeas, kidney beans, lentils, and navy beans, among others.

Whole Grains

- ✓ Barley
- ✓ Buckwheat
- ✓ Bulgur
- ✓ Farro
- ✓ Oats
- ✓ Quinoa
- ✓ Noodles: chow mein, soba
- ✓ Oats
- ✓ Rice: brown, wild, and so on and so on

Herbs & Spices in general

- ✓ Basil

✓ Bay leaves

✓ Chili powder

✓ Chives

✓ Cilantro

✓ Cinnamon

✓ Coriander

✓ Cumin

✓ Curry powder

✓ Dill

✓ Fennel

✓ Fennell

✓ Basil

✓ Bay leaves

✓ Chili powder

✓ Chives

✓ Cilantro

✓ Cinnamon

✓ Coriander

✓ Cumin

✓ Ginger

✓ Mint

✓ Nutmeg

✓ Oregano

✓ Paprika

✓ Parsley

✓ Pepper

✓ Red pepper flakes

✓ Sea salt

✓ Thyme

✓ Garlic/garlic powder

The following are examples of sweeteners: honey, maple syrup, molasses, and pure vanilla essence

Other

✓ Baking powder

✓ Baking soda

✓ Cajun seasoning

✓ Cayenne pepper

✓ Cloves

✓ Cocoa powder

✓ Coffee

✓ Cooking spray

- ✓ Corn taco shells

- ✓ Mustard made using Dijon mustard

- ✓ Flour and alternative flours such as almond flour and cornstarch, among others

- ✓ Hoisin sauce

- ✓ Spicy chili oil

- ✓ Traditional Japanese miso

- ✓ Oyster sauce

- ✓ Protein powder

- ✓ Soy sauce alternatives: tamari sauce or coconut aminos

- ✓ Tea: green

- ✓ Unsweetened nut and seed butter such as almond butter, peanut butter, sunflower seed butter, and so on

- ✓ Vinegar such as apple cider vinegar, balsamic vinegar, rice vinegar, and white wine vinegar

- ✓ Vinegaris made from other grains such as rice

- ✓ Bread made with whole grains or multiple grains

- ✓ Pitas made with whole wheat

- ✓ Tortillas made with whole wheat

- ✓ Worcestershire sauce

REFRIGERATOR AND FREEZER ESSENTIALS

Fruits

- ✓ Cherries
- ✓ Dates;
- ✓ Lemons;
- ✓ Limes;
- ✓ Apples;
- ✓ Apple Juice;
- ✓ Apple Sauce;
- ✓ Bananas; Berries;
- ✓ Blackberries;
- ✓ Blueberries;
- ✓ Raspberries;
- ✓ Strawberries; etc.;
- ✓ Mangoes
- ✓ Nectarines
- ✓ Oranges
- ✓ Peaches

- ✓ Pears
- ✓ Pears
- ✓ Peaches
- ✓ Mangoes

Vegetables

- ✓ Artichoke hearts
- ✓ Asparagus
- ✓ Bean sprouts
- ✓ Bok choy
- ✓ Broccoli
- ✓ Cabbage: red, green, Napa
- ✓ Cauliflower
- ✓ Celeriac
- ✓ Celery
- ✓ Corn
- ✓ Cucumber
- ✓ Edamame
- ✓ Eggplant
- ✓ Fennel

- ✓ Green beans
- ✓ Green peas
- ✓ Greens: chard, collard greens, kale, mustard greens, spinach, and many others
- ✓ Jalapeno
- ✓ Jicama
- ✓ Leeks
- ✓ Onions, including yellow, sweet, and red varieties
- ✓ Peppers in many colors, including green, yellow, orange, and red Pumpkin and radishes both count.
- ✓ Root vegetables such as beets, carrots, parsnips, potatoes, and sweet potatoes;
- ✓ scallions; snow peas; squash such as acorn squash and butternut squash; tomatoes in various forms such as cherry, diced, crushed, paste, and stewed; zucchini

Meats and Proteins

- ✓ Beef products such as ground beef and Canadian bacon;
- ✓ Eggs;
- ✓ Pork; Poultry products such as chicken and turkey;
- ✓ Shellfish and freshwater fish such as shrimp, haddock, trout, salmon, and so on;
- ✓ Tofu

Products Derived from Milk and Other Dairy Alternatives

- ✓ Buttermilk
- ✓ Cheese (including blue cheese, feta, Parmesan, and ricotta);
- ✓ Cottage cheese
- ✓ Kefir
- ✓ Milk
- ✓ Milk substitutes (including almond, cashew, coconut, oat, rice, and soy, among others);
- ✓ Sour cream
- ✓ Greek yogurt and regular yogurt

First Week

I always remind my customers that they need to take one step before they can take two. Therefore I want to offer my congratulations to you as you get ready to take the first step in your journey: week 1.

The first week is all about adjusting to new circumstances, starting again, and confronting the unknown. Either you want to attempt fasting for the first time in a method that is organized, or you are looking to experiment with a new style of fasting.

Meal plans and other instructions that are pretty detailed are supplied for each and every form of fasting. I want to urge you to pay attention to what your body is telling you and to speak openly and honestly about how you are feeling. If you feel as if you need to, you shouldn't be scared to skip a day of your fast or convert to a lighter kind of fasting.

The adaptability of the 12:12 diet makes it possible to have a day of eating that is highly regular while still working toward the objective of achieving a fasting time of 12 hours between your final meal of one day and your first bite of the following day.

12:12 Meal Plan

It contains 12 hours of fasting and 12 hours of eating with three meals per day.

	Breakfast	Lunch	Dinner
Monday	A Porridge Made of Various Grains, Served with Pear and Apple	Asian Grilled Chicken Breasts	Turkey and Vegetable Stew

Tuesday	Ricotta-Oatmeal Pancakes	Wild Rice–Spinach Stew	Kale-Beef Rolls
Wednesday	Delicious Breakfast Casserole Made with Spicy Panzanella	Stuffed peppers with beef and farro	Noodle Salad with Pecan-Tofu and Pecan Crunch
Thursday	Smoothie with Blueberries and Green Tea	Peaches, Sweet Potatoes, and Chicken	Chicken and Bulgur in a Skillet
Friday	Scrambled Tofu, Avocado, and Roasted Red Peppers	A Sweet Potato and Parsnip Frittata	Black Bean & Sun-Dried Tomato Quesadillas
Saturday	Shrimp-Kale Omelet	Rustic Beef & Cabbage Stew	Mediterranean Fish Tacos
Sunday	Baked Cinnamon-Orange French Toast	Broccoli-Beef Stir-Fry with Black Bean Sauce	Classic Roasted Vegetables with Nutmeg

16:8 Meal Plan

It contains 16 hours of fasting time and 8 hours of

eating time with two meals per day.

	Breakfast	Lunch	Dinner
Monday	FAST	Asian Grilled Chicken Breasts	Turkey and Vegetable Stew
Tuesday	FAST	Wild Rice–Spinach Stew	Kale-Beef Rolls
Wednesday	FAST	Stuffed peppers with beef and farro	Noodle Salad with Pecan-Tofu and Pecan Crunch
Thursday	FAST	Peaches, Sweet Potatoes, and Chicken	Chicken and Bulgur in a Skillet

Friday	FAST	A Sweet Potato and Parsnip Frittata	Black Bean & Sun-Dried Tomato Quesadillas
Saturday	FAST	Rustic Beef & Cabbage Stew	Mediterranean Fish Tacos
Sunday	FAST	Broccoli-Beef Stir-Fry with Black Bean Sauce	Classic Roasted Vegetables with Nutmeg

OMAD Meal Plan

It contains 22 hours to 23 hours of fasting time and 1 to 2 hours of eating time with one meal per day.

	Breakfast	Lunch	Dinner
Monday	FAST	FAST	Turkey and Vegetable Stew
Tuesday	FAST	FAST	Kale-Beef Rolls
Wednesday	FAST	FAST	Noodle Salad with Pecan-Tofu and Pecan Crunch
Thursday	FAST	FAST	Chicken and Bulgur in a Skillet
Friday	FAST	FAST	Black Bean & Sun- Dried Tomato Quesadillas
Saturday	FAST	FAST	Mediterranean Fish Tacos
Sunday	FAST	FAST	Classic Roasted Vegetables with Nutmeg

Second Week

Welcome to week 2!

There is awaiting you an exciting new dish that combines many others!

The focus of week 2 is on gaining new knowledge, engaging in self-reflection, and making adjustments as a result of the previous week's activities. Have you had a good experience with the method of fasting that you chose? If that's not the case, I hope you acquired some helpful insight into which kind of fasting could be more appropriate for you.

You shouldn't be scared to make adjustments to your method of fasting or to try something completely new. In the grand scheme of things, one week will not determine very much. The same is true for the exercises you do.

You will be given a brand-new meal plan to follow along with entirely original recipes beginning with the second week of the program.

My money is on the fact that you are finding the meals you eat after breaking your fast to be more satisfying than the meals you eat on a regular basis, and I anticipate that this trend will continue over the following week.

12:12 Meal Plan

It contains 12 hours of fasting and 12 hours of eating with three meals per day.

	Breakfast	Lunch	Dinner
Monday	Date-Fennel Smoothie	Baked Chicken Breasts with Butternut Squash–Pear Salsa	Roasted Pork Chops with Chickpea–Cherry Tomato Salsa

Tuesday	Mixed Grain Porridge with Pear & Maple	Market Bulgur-Chicken Skillet	Pearl Barley–Turkey Soup
Wednesday	Fruit & Nut Yogurt Parfait	Rich Pork Stroganoff	Broiled Beef Tenderloin with Maple Barbecue Sauce
Thursday	Creamy Mango-Jicama Smoothie	Pumpkin-Kale Tortilla	Wraps Salmon–Navy Bean Salad
Friday	Almond Butter–Quinoa Smoothie	Honey Sesame Salmon with Bok Choy	Rich Pork Stroganoff
Saturday	Shrimp-Kale OmeletBaked Egg & Herb Portobello	Mushrooms Pork Tenderloin	Medallions with Herb Sauce Cajun-Style Fish-Tomato Stew
Sunday	Classic Eggs & Canadian Bacon	Traditional Falafel Pockets	Chopped Chicken– Brown Rice Salad

16:8 Meal Plan

It contains 16 hours of fasting time and 8 hours of

eating time with two meals per day.

	Breakfast	**Lunch**	**Dinner**
Monday	FAST	Baked Chicken Breasts with Butternut Squash–Pear Salsa	Roasted Pork Chops with Chickpea– Cherry Tomato Salsa
Tuesday	FAST	Market Bulgur- Chicken Skillet	Pearl Barley– Turkey Soup
Wednesday	FAST	Rich Pork Stroganoff	Broiled Beef

			Tenderloin with Maple Barbecue Sauce
Thursday	FAST	Pumpkin-Kale Tortilla	Wraps Salmon– Navy Bean Salad
Friday	FAST	Honey Sesame Salmon with Bok Choy	Rich Pork Stroganoff
Saturday	FAST	Mushrooms Pork Tenderloin	Medallions with Herb Sauce Cajun-Style Fish- Tomato Stew
Sunday	FAST	Traditional Falafel Pockets	Chopped Chicken– Brown Rice Salad

OMAD Meal Plan

It contains 22 hours to 23 hours of fasting time and 1 to 2 hours of eating time with one meal per day.

	Breakfast	Lunch	Dinner
Monday	FAST	FAST	Roasted Pork Chops with Chickpea–Cherry Tomato Salsa
Tuesday	FAST	FAST	Pearl Barley–Turkey Soup
Wednesday	FAST	FAST	Broiled Beef Tenderloin with Maple Barbecue Sauce
Thursday	FAST	FAST	Wraps Salmon–Navy Bean Salad
Friday	FAST	FAST	Rich Pork Stroganoff
Saturday	FAST	FAST	Medallions with Herb Sauce Cajun-Style Fish- Tomato Stew
Sunday	FAST	FAST	Chopped Chicken–Brown Rice Salad

Third Week

I cannot tell you how excited I am to welcome you to week 3!

Although you are about to reach the conclusion of one phase of your adventure via intermittent fasting, it is my sincere desire that this 21-day process is only the beginning for you.

We hope that at this time, you have some respect for how flexible fasting can be. Whether you discovered a sort of fasting that you love during week one, or you are still getting there, we hope that you have some appreciation for how flexible fasting can be. Even if you have adhered to a very tight framework up to this point, it is essential to keep in mind that after this last week, you will have more leeway to experiment with different ways to make fasting work for you. The mouthwatering dishes that have been offered for week three will undoubtedly be of assistance with that. Enjoy!

12:12 Meal Plan

It contains 12 hours of fasting and 12 hours of eating with three meals per day.

	Breakfast	Lunch	Dinner
Monday	Fruit & Nut Yogurt Parfait	Fiery Pork Lettuce Wraps	Grain-&-Tofu-Stuffed Eggplant with Tahini
Tuesday	Shrimp–Kale Omelet	Bulgur Lettuce Tacos	Chicken & Artichoke Heart Pita Pizza
Wednesday	Blueberry–Green Tea Smoothie	Chopped Chicken–Brown Rice Salad	Pan-Seared Trout with Dill & Leeks
Thursday	Baked Egg & Herb	Mediterranean Fish	Tofu Moussaka

	Portobello Mushrooms	Tacos	
Friday	Mixed Grain Porridge with Pear & Maple	Edamame Mixed Green Salad with Berries	Pork–Bok Choy Chow Mein
Saturday	Ricotta-Oatmeal Pancakes	Pearl Barley–Turkey Soup	Baked Haddock-Mushroom Casserole
Sunday	Classic Eggs & Canadian Bacon Honey	Curried Peanut Vegetable Noodles	Sesame Salmon with Bok Choy

16:8 Meal Plan

It contains 16 hours of fasting time and 8 hours of

eating time with two meals per day.

	Breakfast	Lunch	Dinner
Monday	FAST	Fiery Pork Lettuce Wraps	Grain-&-Tofu-Stuffed Eggplant with Tahini
Tuesday	FAST	Bulgur Lettuce Tacos	Chicken & Artichoke Heart Pita Pizza
Wednesday	FAST	Chopped Chicken– Brown Rice Salad	Pan-Seared Trout with Dill & Leeks
Thursday	FAST	Mediterranean Fish Tacos	Tofu Moussaka
Friday	FAST	Edamame Mixed Green	Pork–Bok Choy Chow

		Salad with Berries	Mein
Saturday	FAST	Pearl Barley–Turkey Soup	Baked Haddock-Mushroom Casserole
Sunday	FAST	Curried Peanut Vegetable Noodles	Sesame Salmon with Bok Choy

OMAD Meal Plan

It contains 22 hours to 23 hours of fasting time and 1 to 2 hours of eating time with one meal per day.

	Breakfast	Lunch	Dinner
Monday	FAST	FAST	Grain-&-Tofu-Stuffed Eggplant with Tahini
Tuesday	FAST	FAST	Chicken & Artichoke Heart Pita Pizza
Wednesday	FAST	FAST	Pan-Seared Trout with Dill & Leeks
Thursday	FAST	FAST	Tofu Moussaka
Friday	FAST	FAST	Pork–Bok Choy Chow Mein
Saturday	FAST	FAST	Baked Haddock-Mushroom Casserole
Sunday	FAST	FAST	Sesame Salmon with Bok Choy

Conclusion

Even while intermittent fasting is often regarded as a healthy and productive way of living as well as a method of eating, there are circumstances in which a person could not benefit the most from adhering to this specific eating plan.

These circumstances include: It is essential for those who are interested in adopting an intermittent fasting diet first to analyze the benefits and drawbacks of this diet, as well as have a look at the particular dangers that have been connected with this method of eating. If the person discovers that they could be on the riskier side of things, then the practice of intermittent fasting might not be the best solution for them. If this is the case, the individual could be best served by choosing an alternate diet that might assist them in accomplishing their particular objectives.

Before beginning to adopt a plan like intermittent fasting in your own life, it is recommended that you first discuss the topic with a medical professional, as is the case with any form of meal plan or alteration to the way you are now adjusting your eating habits. It is in your best interest to select a doctor who is already familiar with both you and your past medical history.

In this way, the doctor will be in a position to determine whether or not you would be a suitable candidate for intermittent fasting and whether or not a different kind of diet might be more appropriate for you.

Before beginning to adhere to a diet that includes periods of intermittent fasting, it is essential for women to get the OK from their primary care provider.

The reason for this is that research has shown that in certain instances, intermittent fasting may have a negative effect on the hormonal balance that naturally exists inside the body of a woman.

In the event that a woman's hormones are not in a state of equilibrium, she runs the risk of experiencing a variety of potentially negative repercussions.

When a woman's hormones are out of whack, she runs the risk of experiencing a number of unpleasant outcomes, some of which include the following:

Developing skin-related issues, such as dry skin, is persistent among women who have an imbalance in hormones inside their bodies. This may lead to a variety of skin-related difficulties.

The appearance of acne is yet another prevalent symptom that may be brought on by this specific issue. [Cause and effect] Skin discolorations are another potential complication that might arise.

All of these things have the potential to adversely affect a woman's mental health, making it more likely that she would develop feelings of insecurity over her physical attractiveness.

Brain fog is another symptom that might appear if a woman's hormones are not functioning normally:

This may be a very distressing problem for the lady, as she may find that she is unable to focus and concentrate, and her memory may also be negatively impacted as a result of the situation. As a direct result of this, the woman's overall productivity will face a significant drop. Keeping this in mind, the quality of their work time will suffer as a result.

An imbalance in a woman's hormone levels may cause a number of unpleasant symptoms, including brain fog, weariness, and repeated instances of the latter, particularly in women. It's possible that fatigue is much worse.

It's possible that the lady may discover that she is perpetually exhausted and has an increased need to sleep.

Mood swings are another symptom that is relatively prevalent among women who have problems with the hormonal balance in their bodies. Swings in one's mood are sometimes accompanied by episodes of worry, tension, and even melancholy in certain people.

Inadequate management of a woman's hormones may sometimes also result in a decrease in her libido, particularly in circumstances when the woman is sexually active.

In the event that the woman's libido is low, she will have no desire to engage in sexual activity with their spouse.

When it comes to incorporating a strategy for intermittent fasting into one's life, those who are afflicted with specific diseases will also need to exercise extreme caution. When it comes to intermittent fasting, adrenal tiredness, preexisting hormonal difficulties, and gastrointestinal troubles are some of the ailments that are regarded to be risk factors for suffering unpleasant consequences from the practice.

People who have a history of eating disorders are also advised to steer clear of the practice of intermittent fasting since it has the potential to produce unfavorable effects.

This is because of the potential for the practice to create undesirable outcomes.

Printed in Great Britain
by Amazon

34249855R00109